Herbal Remedies for Glowing Skin

Natural Home Remedies You Can't Afford to Know!

Disclaimer

No part of this eBook can be spread or reproduced in any form including print, electronic, photocopying, scanning, mechanical or recording without the author's consent.

The remedies mentioned here should not be used if they alter or substitute with your medical therapy without taking your doctor's advice. For certain health problems, consult your physician first before using the recipes in this eBook.

Always check with your physician to avoid any adverse effects that could rise from the usage of these recipes if you have an existing medical condition, or if you are pregnant or nursing.

Some herbs can also interact with your medical prescriptions including antidepressants and the Pill. Furthermore, if thinking of using any of the skin balms, always do a 24-hour skin test before using to avoid any allergic reactions from the ingredients. It is understood that the reader claims responsibility for their own actions.

All information, recipes and ideas presented here are for educational purposes only. The author cannot be held responsible for any personal or commercial damage caused by misinterpretation of information or improper use of the details in this eBook.

Summary

Every year people spend heaps of money on spas getting treatments for radiant, glowing and flawless skin. All these treatments and visits to spas are getting expensive with the passage of time. It appears a waste of money to spend so much on chemical based treatments in spas when you can achieve better results by home remedies.

Are you shocked? Well don't be. Herbal and home remedies have been among us for centuries and women in all eras have always longed for radiant glowing skin. Back in time when these spas and treatments weren't here, women used to achieve beautiful glowing skin with help of these home remedies.

This eBook will tell you about:

1. How to use simple ingredients from the kitchen to achieve glowing skin.
2. Step by step recipes for a home made mask according to oily and dry skin types.
3. Results of ingredients and the impact they will have on your skin.

When you finish reading this eBook you will have all the information that you need about home remedies to make your skin glowing and radiant. However, it is advised that you make sure that you are not allergic to any ingredient mentioned in the recipes. Before applying any mask, make sure you perform a patch test 24 hours before.

So what are you waiting for? Sit back, relax and plunge into the world of home remedies.

Contents

Introduction

Every day our skin has to tolerate so much! From harsh chemicals of makeup, beauty products, heat, pollution and what not? With all that to tolerate our skin needs some revival. It needs care to make it look beautiful, glowing and refreshing.

Indeed, there are several products available in the market that promise to rid you of all the skin problems and issues that you have ever had. While these beauty products are useful in the long run they harm your skin too. In some cases excessive use of these chemicals can cause early aging of the skin. Then you will have to use anti-aging products. It is a circle of using more chemical products to solve the issues that other chemical products have created in the first place. Now isn't it bizarre?

For this exact reason there exist home remedies. Yes! You read it right. Home remedies have been around us always. Our mother, grandmothers and even grand grandmothers have been making use of home remedies and secret ingredients in their kitchen to make their skin appear naturally radiant and beautiful.

There are home remedies for all skin types. The benefits of using home remedies to look beautiful are that they comprise of all natural products. They are not going to harm your skin unless you are allergic to any of the ingredients. It is advised that you do a patch test before using any home remedy, to avoid any sort of complication later on.

First things first, to get naturally glowing skin, you need to get rid of all the problems of your skin. Issues like acne, black heads, white heads, dark spots, so on and so forth. In this eBook you will read all about sorts of home remedies that you need to know to get a glowing, beautiful, younger looking healthy skin.

Bleach for Naturally Glowing Skin

Your face represents you and distinguishes you from and among the crowd. To have glowing skin, what better home remedy will there be other than bleach? By the word bleach our first instinct is "Yikes! It is going to burn" Well not any more. With natural bleaching options available why would you go for chemical products?

Bleach with Lemon Juice

Lemon has natural bleaching agents; it removes dirt and naturally lightens your skin tone and bleaches your face.

Ingredients

7-8 Fresh Lemons

1 tablespoon Honey

Water

Process:

Cut the lemons in halves and squeeze the juice in a clean bowl. Add some water to the lemon juice and dilute it. Take a cotton ball, dip it in the diluted solution and apply it gently on your face. Don't rub it. Gently apply it all over your face and wash your face with water after 10 minutes.

Effect:

Lemon will remove all the dirt and will lighten your skin tone and allows your skin to breath.

Bleach with Yogurt

Nothing feels more relaxing than a good mask after a long tiring week.

Ingredients:

1 tablespoon Fresh Tomato Juice

1 tablespoon Yogurt

1 tablespoon Oatmeal

Process:

Mix all of the ingredients in a clean bowl and make a fine paste. Apply this mask after cleansing your skin and allow it dry for good 10-15 minutes.

Effects:

This mask is best for all skin types. Yogurt will significantly reduce any trace of blemishes and will moisturize your skin, making it look and feel supple.

Yogurt also lightens your tone and acts as a natural bleach.

Say Bye-Bye to Acne

The biggest problem in anyone's life can be pimples. Isn't it annoying when suddenly a pimple on your face becomes the center of attention at a gathering? They hide the true beauty of your face and in extreme cases can even cause dull complexion.

There can be several reasons for pimples. It can be hormonal or improper diet or may be due to your skin type. People with oily skin usually face issues of pimples. It is integral to know why you are facing acne. However here are some home remedies for you which work like magic for pimples.

Use Yogurt and Orange Peel for Blemishes and Acne

Orange is high in vitamin C concentration and it is a vital ingredient for fresh skin.

Ingredients

Orange Peels

Yogurt

Process:

Put the orange peel on newspaper and leave it out to dry. Orange peels will take approximately a day or two to dry. But make sure to keep them in a warm dry place. When they are dried grind them to a powdered form and store the powder in an air tight jar.

Mix one tablespoon of orange peel powder with 1 tablespoon or yogurt and make a paste. Apply the paste on your face with the help of a brush or fingers and let it dry. Use some water and massage your face for a few minutes before washing it off with water. Don't rub vigorously if you have acne. Be gentle.

Effect:

Orange will make all the dark spots and blemishes go away. You can repeat the process 2-3 times a week for better results.

Use of Tomato Pulp

Tomato is a bit acidic in nature and if you apply tomato juice or its pulp, the vitamins K, C and A present in the fruit helps in drying up the pimple. With frequent use it can help you in getting a fair, clear and glowing skin free of acne. It is advised that for better results, apply tomato pulp as a mask on your face.

Use of Garlic

Garlic has the properties of an antibiotic and serves as a cleaning agent on pimples. It kills the germs and helps you in getting rid of the pimples. Cut the garlic and apply its essence on pimples. Don't directly apply garlic as it is hard and can cause bleeding.

Use of Cucumber

It is a general perception that most skin problems are due to oily skin and sebum but what if someone has dry skin and still faces a pimple problem? The problem at times can be dehydration of the skin. You need to properly hydrate your skin to avoid any sort of skin complications. Use of a cucumber mask can be extremely effective in this case.

Ingredients:

1 cucumber

Water

Process:

Grind cucumber into a pulp and add some water to form the consistency of a thick paste. Apply this paste all over your face and your neck and leave it for 30 minutes. Wash your face with warm water.

Effect:

Your skin will feel lighter and supple. Cucumber has a cooling effect and it hydrates your skin.

Use of Olive Oil

Generally acne problems arise due to skin being too oily and the idea that olive oil can help anyone with acne can seem a bit absurd. But it is not. Olive oil can be of great use for people with pimples. Pimples can make your skin appear dry and scaly. A mixture of Olive oil and salt can help your skin to feel moisturized and glowing. Apply the mixture on the affected area and rinse with water.

Use of Lemon Juice

Lemon juice has vitamin C and is high in citric acid concentration. Use of lemon not only helps in drying the pimples/acne it also acts as an antibacterial and reduces the growth of pimples. Vitamin C and citric acid found in the lemon also helps you in getting a glowing skin. Apply it on your face with the help of a cotton ball.

Precautions you need to take when applying; don't rub the area after application and wash it gently afterwards. Also avoid coming in direct contact with sun as it can cause darkening of your skin.

Use of Cinnamon with Honey

Honey has all of the abilities and properties of a good antibacterial. The use of honey prevents the growth of acne and blemishes and helps you in maintaining a flawless and radiant skin.

Honey if used in combination with cinnamon can do wonders for people with acne problems. Cinnamon stick has oils that are essential for our skin. It is the key ingredient of several acne treatment creams. A mask of honey with cinnamon can rejuvenate your skin, kill the bacteria and provide the moisture your skin might have lost due to the acne problem.

Ingredients:

Cinnamon sticks

Honey

Process:

Put some water in a boiling pan and let it boil. Add 2 cinnamon sticks and a tablespoon of honey and stir until the water is of honey color. Put the pan aside and allow the mixture to cool. Apply the solution on your face with a cotton ball and allow it to dry. Wash it with lukewarm water.

Use of Lavender Oil

Make it a habit. Every time you have a blemish or acne outbreak, take lavender oil on your finger tip and massage it on the blemish. It will wipe out the pimples.

You can even add a bit of lavender oil while taking the steam and then gently wipe off the dirt of your face. It will open your pores and allow your skin to breathe. Clean pores means no pimples.

Use of Iced-Tea Cubes

Iced-tea is an antioxidant. It helps to better the circulation of oxygen in your blood and helps in detoxification of blood. This eventually helps in better, healthier and glowing skin. Consumption of Iced-Tea or green tea is recommended if you want to have clear skin.

However as far as the home remedies is concerned, you can freeze the iced-tea in cubes and gently massage it on your face. You can make it a ritual and do it regularly after being exposed to sun.

Use of Strawberries

Pimples are not always with puss, at times they are just red and hurt. For such pimples strawberries are extremely effective. Cut the top of the strawberries and rub the moist part on your pimples. This will give them a cooling effect. Gently massage it on the pimples and give it a rest for a good 30 minutes and then wash thoroughly. Oh and you can still eat the strawberries.

Use of Neem Tree Leaves

Call them Neem tree leaves or magical leaves. Because of their amazing healing and antiseptic powers, you can name them anything you like. Neem tree is known and famous for helping people in getting rid of acne and pimples. You can use Neem in a number of ways to get rid of the pimples.

At times it happens that there is only one pimple on your face and the next thing you know they just keep popping up. It can at times be due to bacterial growth. In this case Neem leaves can help you in a number of ways.

1. Boil Neem tree leaves in water and then set it aside and allow it to cool. Fill a spray bottle. If you have acne or not. Before applying makeup, or going to bed or after washing your face, spray the water all over your face and allow it dry. Don't wash your face afterwards. It will act as an antibacterial tonic and will prevent further growth of acne due to sebum or excess oil.
2. Neem Oil also has magical effects when it comes to solving the pimple issues. Apply the Neem oil directly to the blemishes with a cotton ball, before going to bed. Wash your face in the morning with water.
3. Neem powder is easily available in the market. But if you can't find it, crush the neem leaves and make a paste with water. Apply the paste on the pimples and allow it to dry. When dry wash it with lukewarm water. If you have puss pimples then it will help in drying them and prevent them from leaving marks.

Miracle of Rose Water

At times most acne problems arise due to sebum. To prevent oily skin and sebum on your face, always keep rose water in a spray bottle with you. Spray rose water on your face and either wipe it with a tissue gently or allow it dry. It will freshen up your face and will prevent blemishes from popping up.

If you have blemishes, mix a tablespoon of lemon juice in rose water and apply it directly on the blemishes. The antibacterial property of lemon will prevent any new bacterial growth and rose water will refresh your skin and give a cooling and calm effect to your skin.

Skin Lightening Remedies for a Glowing Skin

Make it a point that 'healthy skin is glowing skin'. Sometimes prolonged exposure to sun, heat and pollution can cause your skin to look dull and dark. This can cause your natural skin color to fade.

Even though several skin lightening creams and treatments are available in the market, they are only good as long as you keep using them. The result of these products doesn't last long.

However if you want your skin to always look lighter, healthier and glowing then the following remedies will be of great use to you.

1. Lemon

Lemon is one fruit that has many benefits and is utilized in several home remedies. Cut a lemon into halves and directly apply on the parts of your body that has been exposed to sun. Their however is one precautionary measure that you have to take. When you have applied lemon juice on your skin, avoid coming in contact with direct heat or sunlight.

2. Orange

Orange is yet another useful fruit and helps in lightening your skin tone. You can use orange juice and apply it all over your face and let it dry for 10-15 minutes. The orange juice will act as a natural toner.

3. Milk

Lactic Acid in milk is extremely helpful in lightening the tone of your skin. It works as a toner for all skin types. You can apply it all over your face after cleansing or before going to bed. Make sure that the milk you apply on your face is not boiled; raw milk is very helpful and beneficial for skin lightening.

a. Milk Cream

Milk cream is also part of milk and has similar moisturizing and lightening effects on your skin. A face mask of milk cream and Saffron helps in lightening your skin and leaves your skin smooth, supple and glowing.

Ingredients:

1 tablespoon Milk cream

Few strands of Saffron

Process:

Mix Saffron in milk cream and make a paste. Apply the paste on your face and let it dry for an hour. Spray rose water on your face and then massage your face for a few minutes before washing the mask with water.

4. Turmeric Powder

Turmeric powder can do wonders when it comes to skin lightening. Turmeric has long been used as an antiseptic and a beauty product. It has many benefits and should always be kept at home.

Turmeric powder can give you astonishing results if applied in combination with other ingredients.

a. Turmeric and Orange Juice:

Turmeric powder in orange juice and make a fine paste. Apply the paste all over your face with a gentle hand, don't rub it. Apply it on your face before going to bed and remove it the next morning with help of warm water. Make sure you don't stain your pillow cover.

b. Turmeric and Lemon:

Mix lemon juice with a pinch of turmeric powder. Apply it all over your face as a tonic and wash it after half an hour. You will be amazed how glowing your skin will get.

c. Turmeric and Tomatoes:

Take a medium sized tomato blend it into a puree. Add 4 tablespoon of lemon juice and a pinch of turmeric powder and apply it on your face as a mask. Allow it to dry and wash it after 30 minutes.

5. Aloe Vera

Aloe Vera works like magic with all skin types. It is like a magic potion that has the tendency to solve all the skin problems that you can list.

Cut the Aloe Vera and extract the gel from the leaves' center into a bowl. Mash it further with the help of a spoon/fork and apply it generously on your face. Gently massage with the gel on your face for few minutes and then allow it to dry. Wash it after an hour or so.

Aloe Vera will help in reviving your natural skin tone and will reduce the effects of sun and heat.

6. Honey

Honey is the best thing that can happen to the world of beauty and health care. It is the key ingredient of most of your beauty products.

You can apply honey directly on your face and remove it after a couple of hours. It will make your skin glow and feel moisturized.

Honey also gives great results if used in combination with other ingredients like Olive oil and lemon. Honey will help in removing dead cells and allow your skin to breathe and feel fresh again!

7. Gram Flour

If you think whitening creams can lighten your skin tone, then you haven't tried gram flour yet. It is one of the simplest and easiest ingredients that work like magic. Apart from other benefits, gram flour masks can lighten your skin tone.

Ingredient:

1 tablespoon gram flour

Rose water

Process:

Mix gram flour in rose water and make a thick paste. Apply it all over your face and neck and allow it to dry. Wash it with water and massage thoroughly.

Herbal Home Remedies for Oily Skin:

Sebum protects your skin, but when it accumulates in abundance it makes your skin oily. How irritating it is that no amount of makeup can help you in hiding the extra oil on your T-zone. Then again there are women who have been using several cosmetic products for years but even they aren't of great help. These products might help you in oil-controlling but they also make your skin look darker. Either way you lose the freshness of your skin.

Oily skin is not a skin type; it is more of a skin condition. Your skin may become oily due to hormonal changes in your teens or during menstrual cycle or menopause or during pregnancy in women where as in men it can be due to hormonal changes as well.

But having oily skin is not all that bad. The fun fact about people with oily skin is that they tend to look younger and their aging starts late compared to people with dry skin. Here are few home remedies that will help you in getting rid of the oil on your face and make it look fresh and glowing.

Massage Your Face:

Fine Grain Masks

Gram flour has the tendency to absorb oil. Using a gram flour face mask will help you in getting rid of the excessive oil on your face that clogs up the pores.

Ingredients:

2 tablespoon dry oats powder

Witch Hazel

Rose Water

Process:

Mix the ingredients well and form a paste of thick consistency. Apply it all over your face and allow the mask to dry. Dip a cotton ball in the rose water and remove the mask with it. Spray rose water on your face and allow it dry.

Butter Milk Massage:

2-3 times a week, apply buttermilk on your face and massage it with finger tips. Buttermilk has the acidic properties that help in cleaning the pores and removing the dead skin, leaving your skin glowing. Butter milk is even a good remedy to tighten your skin and cleansing.

Give it a rest after massage and then rinse thoroughly.

Home Made Masks

Every month you spend a lot of money for getting your facial done and soothing masks at the spa. With little effort at home you can not only save some money you will be able to take care of your skin better at home. These quick masks can be made at home and will help you in curing oily skin and its effects.

Mud Masks:

Mud masks or commonly known as clay masks are extremely useful when it comes to getting rid of the grease and oil on the skin. They are extremely effective in removing the impurities. These mud masks are easily available on the natural or herbal stores. You can use French clay mud, fuller's earth, volcanic mud, black mud or alpine moor mud. Don't forget to do a patch test before you apply it on your face, you may be allergic to one or other type of the mud.

Ingredients:

2 full tablespoons of French clay mud/Fuller's earth/volcanic mud/Black mud/Alpine moor mud

Rose Water (To make paste)

Process:

Make a fine paste using the ingredients and apply it on your face with the help of a brush. Make sure you cover every inch of your face with enough paste. Allow it to dry and keep your face straight. Remember the rule, No laughing or smiling.

These mud masks not only remove the oil and grease from your skin but they are also helpful in skin tightening and getting rid of the wrinkles and fine lines and leaving a glowing fresh skin for you to cherish.

Egg-White Masks:

Use of an egg white mask is very ancient. They are extremely effective when it comes to oil controlling. It also helps in skin tightening and removes signs of aging. It will also unclog the pores.

Ingredients:

1 Egg white

1 tablespoon honey

1 tablespoon of flour

Process:

Mix the entire ingredients well and form a thick paste. Apply it all over your face and neck and give it a rest for some time. When the mask dries, rinse thoroughly with lukewarm water.

Fruit Masks

Fruits masks are always good to use when it comes to oil controlling. It is best to make use of these face masks at home instead of getting expensive fruit facials at the spa.

Mango Mask

Take one medium mango's flesh in a clean bowl and mash it into pulp with the help of a fork or grind it. Apply the pulp all over your face for 20-25 minutes and then remove it. Wash thoroughly with water.

Apple and Honey Mask

Remove the seeds of an apple and grind it into a pulp then add 4 tablespoons of honey and mix well until it starts to look like a paste. Apply it on your face. Leave it for about 10-15 minutes and then wash it thoroughly.

Wheat Flour Mask

Take 3 tablespoons of wheat flour and make a paste with water or rose water. Apply it all over your face. Make sure you apply using upward strokes. Let it dry and wash your face with lukewarm water. Apply rose water or witch hazel on your face afterwards.

Milk and Cucumber Mask

Take one cucumber and grind it well to extract the cucumber juice from pulp and mix with milk. Apply the mixture all over your face with the help of a cotton ball and allow it to dry. It will give you a cooling and soothing effect and will also make your skin glow.

Fenugreek Seeds' Mask

The Fenugreek mask will act as an exfoliating agent for oily skin. It also helps in removing black heads and is even useful in cases of eczema.

Keep 2-3 tablespoons of fenugreek seeds in water and soak it for at least 12 hours. Crush and grind the seeds to a paste and apply it all over your face and neck. When it's dried massage your face with gentle hands and dust off the mask. Wash your face thoroughly afterwards.

Make Natural Toner:

After scrubbing and applying face masks, your pores are open and dust and dirt will clog the pores if you don't take care of them. After you are done with your facial and mask, it is advised to apply toner to close the pores and keep them from clogging. There are several products available in the market but you can always make your own toner at home. Because, what is better than a natural way to maintain your beauty.

Witch Hazel Toner

Witch hazel works like magic when it comes to closing up your pores. You can even use it in the face masks. Apply witch hazel all over your face after you wash, scrub or cleanse your face. Witch Hazel has acerbic properties. It cuts off the oil and prevents oil from accumulating on your face by tightening the pores.

Sage, Yarrow and Peppermint Toner

Sage, yarrow and peppermint are natural herbs. They have acerbic and toning properties. You can make a toner with these herbs at home and apply it on your face daily for better results.

Ingredients:

1 tablespoon Sage

1 tablespoon Yarrow

1 tablespoon Peppermint

1 cup Water

Process:

Put all the herbs in a cup and pour hot boiling water on it and cover the cup for half an hour. When cool, filter the herbs from the water and store it in a spray bottle. The toner can last for at least 3-4 days if stored in the fridge.

Hyssop Toner

Hyssop is also an extremely useful herb and was used as an agent to gain fair and glowing complexion in ancient times. Toner made from Hyssop will help in keeping the oil and sebum from accumulating on your skin.

Ingredients:

1 Tablespoon of Hyssop Herb

1 Cup Water

Process:

Boil water in a pan and add the hyssop herb to it. Turn off the stove and cover the pan. Set aside and let it cool. Filter the herbs from the water and store it in a spray bottle. Apply daily for best results.

Lavender Oil:

Lavender and Orange Bud oil (Commonly known as Neroli Oil) are extremely helpful in toning and cleansing of the face. You can use a mixture of these 2 as a toner after washing your face daily. You can spray the mixture on your face multiple times for a refreshing look.

Getting Rid of Whiteheads

Whiteheads are the remnants of dirt and dead skin that clogs up in the pores of your skin and turns into pimples later on. Getting rid of whiteheads is equally important to getting rid of pimples. Here are a couple of homemade scrubs and masks that will be of great use to you.

Steam:

It gets easier to remove and extract whiteheads with steam. Steam softens the whiteheads and helps in easy removal. Soak a towel in warm water and place it on your face. Leave it for some time and then repeat the process at least 5-6 times in one sitting.

Rub the towel all over your face with firm pressure; this will help to remove whiteheads from your face.

Scrub:

Scrub of wheat flour and oatmeal is best for getting rid of whiteheads. Make a paste by using 1 tablespoon of oatmeal and wheat flour and add just enough rose water to form a thick consistency. Scrub well with the mixture for 2-3 minutes then remove it with the help of a wet sponge. This scrub will also remove oil and grease from your skin along with whiteheads.

Cleanse

Milk and lemon cleansers are deemed as one of the best homemade remedies when it comes to removal of whiteheads and reducing the formation of pustules. This remedy will serve as a cleanser.

Ingredients:

1 tablespoon of Lemon juice

2 tablespoons of Milk

1 tablespoon of Salt

Process:

Mix all the ingredients and stir well to form a solution. Apply it all over your face and massage gently for 4-5 minutes. Wipe your face off with the help of a sponge and then wash it with water thoroughly.

Mask:

After cleansing, scrubbing and steaming comes the turn of a mask! Use the following masks to get rid of the whiteheads completely.

Tomato Pulp:

Remove the seeds of tomato and grind the flesh into a thick pulp. Add a tablespoon of honey and apply it all over your face. Leave the mask as it is for 30 minutes and then rinse thoroughly with the help of water.

Toothpaste

It might surprise you a bit but yes, toothpaste can be used as a home remedy to get rid of black and whiteheads alike. Apply toothpaste on your face where blackheads and whiteheads have popped up. Let it dry and then wash it with water.

Potato Mask

Peel a potato and grind it. Add some rose water to turn it into a thick paste and then grind again. Apply the mixture all over your face, allow it to dry and then wash your face with lukewarm water.

Fenugreek Leaves:

Just like Fenugreek seeds, its leaves are of great use too. They are extremely useful in removal of white heads.

Process:

Wash fenugreek leaves and make a paste of them using water. Apply it on your face and massage for 2-3 minutes. Apply it at night before going to bed. Wash it the next morning with lukewarm water. Repeating the process 2-3 times a week will show visible results in just one week.

Herbal Home Remedies for Getting Rid of Blackheads:

Blackheads are the biggest hurdle in the way of achieving a flawless and glowing skin. Blackheads are the result of oily skin. You need to cure the oily skin to get rid of the blackheads. No matter how tempted you are to use your nails to squeeze out the blackheads, it is an extremely unhygienic and unsafe way to deal with blackheads. You might end up hurting yourself.

There are other natural and scrumptious ways to get rid of the oil and blackheads. These yummy ingredients from your kitchen will serve as great home remedies.

Oatmeal Mask:

Ingredients:

1 Tablespoon Oatmeal

1 Tablespoon Oatmeal Paste

1 Tablespoon Lemon Juice

1 Tablespoon Olive Oil

Process:

Mix all the ingredients and make a fine paste. Heat the mix just enough to make it warm. The mixture should be slightly warm so that your skin can tolerate it. Apply it all over your face and neck with the help of a brush. Give it a rest for some time. This mask will absorb oil from your face and unclog your pores and remove blackheads.

Always make sure that you are not allergic to any or all of the natural products. Perform a patch test before applying all over your face.

Almond Mask

Scrubs are extremely helpful when it comes to getting rid of clogged pores and blackheads. Almond and chickpea scrub will be a good home remedy for getting rid of blackheads. Mix a spoon full of crushed almonds and chickpea flour with a few drops of rose water.

Apply it on your face and scrub it gently with fingers for 3-4 minutes. It will extract out the blackheads and will unclog the pores.

Turmeric Powder and Coriander Leaves Mask

Coriander leaves have so many benefits. One of them is that it helps you in getting rid of blackheads and turmeric will lighten up your skin tone and unclog pores. Crush coriander leaves and mix a tablespoon of turmeric powder in it. Add just enough water to form a paste and apply it on your face and scrub well for 2-3 minutes.

Lemon and Sugar Scrub

Take one tablespoon of sugar and add 1 tablespoon of lemon juice to it. Stir well and form a mixture. Apply it all over your face and scrub gently for 2-3 minutes.

Baking Soda

Baking soda can be used for a lot of purposes, including for removal of blackheads. Apply a mixture of baking soda and rose water on your face. Leave it for 15-20 minutes and then wash it off while gently massaging your face.

Cinnamon and Honey

Cinnamon is extremely effective when it comes to easy removal of blackheads. A face mask prepared with cinnamon, lemon juice and honey helps in unclogging the pores and removes dirt and excess oil from your face.
Ingredients:
2 Tablespoons of Lemon Juice
1 Tablespoon of Honey
1 Tablespoon of Cinnamon Powder
Process:
Mix the ingredients and form a thick paste. Apply the paste on the areas where blackheads have appeared. Let it sit like that for a good 20 minutes and allow it to dry. Wipe your face with the help of a wet sponge and then wash your face thoroughly with lukewarm water.
You can even apply it on your face before going to bed and wash your face the next morning with lukewarm water.

Quick Home Remedies to Remove Black and Whiteheads

a. Almond and Chickpea Mask

Grind almond to a fine paste. Take 1 teaspoon of almond powder and 1 teaspoon of chickpea flour. Add rose water to it and apply it all over your face. Once you do that allow it to dry. When it is dry, spray some rose water on your face and massage your face with it. Especially the areas in which black and whiteheads have appeared.

b. Honey and Almond Mask

Crush almond into semi powder form take a teaspoon of almond powder and 1 tablespoon of honey and make a paste. Add some rose water if you think the consistency of the mixture is too thick. Apply the mixture on your face and gently massage your face on your cheeks, chin and nose. Wash your face after the massage with lukewarm water.

c. Yogurt and Lemon Paste

Take 2 spoons full of yogurt and add 1 Tablespoon of lemon juice to it. Mix well and form a paste. Apply the paste all over your face thoroughly and massage until it is completely absorbed. Wash your face thoroughly with lukewarm water. This mixture will not only help you in getting rid of blackheads but it will also unclog the pores, allowing your skin to breathe.

d. Aloe Vera

Apply Aloe Vera gel on the area where blackheads have appeared. Gently massage with the gel on the area with blackheads.

e. Steam

It is a common misconception that if you steam regularly your pores will stay open and this will result in pimples. This is a myth. It is advised that you steam your face twice a week. Steaming opens your pores and makes it easier for you to remove the blackheads and whiteheads. But don't forget to apply toner after cleansing and scrubbing.

f. Rose Water

Make it a habit. Keep rose water in your bag in a spray bottle. Spray your face with it several times a day. It not only makes your face feel refreshed but it also prevents oil from accumulating on your skin and resulting in black and whiteheads.

g. Nutmeg Powder

Nutmeg has the properties of a scrub. Make a fine paste using 1 Tablespoon of nutmeg and milk. Apply it all over your face and neck. Massage your face gently, especially the areas with black and whiteheads. The combination of these two provides the nourishment your skin requires while removing the black and whiteheads.

Herbal Home Remedies for Dry Skin:

Taking care of oily skin is difficult but taking care of dry skin is equally important. Dry skin sufferers don't face problems like accumulation of sebum and oil on their face. However, if they don't take good care of their skin, dry skin is more likely to show early aging signs and can face serious skin problems.

On a daily basis our skin has to go through a lot. Even the slightest change in weather leaves its marks on dry skin. These home remedies don't take longer than 10-20 minutes to prepare. Your skin requires attention and care. By following a few quick tips and tricks at home you can take good care of dry skin and have a flawless, healthy and glowing skin.

Homemade Masks:

Masks for dry skin should be those which help in regaining the moisture of your skin and make it look supple and nourished. Certain fruits and dry fruits have natural essential oils in them. If used properly they will provide the natural nourishment, essential oils and moisture your skin may have lost due to use of harsh chemicals and pollution.

Banana Mask

Take one medium sized banana and mash it into a paste with the help of a fork or grind it. Add 1-2 Tablespoons of honey to form a paste and mix well. Apply the paste on your face and spread it well while gently massaging your face. Leave it like that for 10 minutes and then wash your face thoroughly with water.

Milk and Peanuts Mask

Grind milk and 10-12 peanuts to form a thick consistency paste. Apply it all over your face and massage for 2-3 minutes. Allow it to dry and then wash your face with the help of water. Apply rose water on your face afterwards.

Milk Cream and Oil Mask

Take one Tablespoon of Milk cream and half a Tablespoon of Olive oil and a dash of turmeric powder. Mix well and form a paste. Apply it all over your face and massage gently. Apply all the paste to your skin. Clean your face with a wet sponge and then wash your face with water thoroughly. You can even replace olive oil with coconut oil.

This mixture will rejuvenate your skin and provide it with the moisture it requires to look fresh, young and glowing.

Moisturize to Prevent the Skin from Getting Dry and Scaly

Moisturizing is to dry skin as water is to life. Dry skin usually appears extremely unappealing and leaves an impression as if you don't care about your looks. Your face represents you and it is integral to look after your skin, especially if it is dry.

You can moisturize your skin by a number of ways. The good part about having dry skin is that you don't have to worry about remedies which will accumulate oil on your skin unlike people with oily skin.

Avocado Moisturizer

Avocado has essential oils that rejuvenates and repairs your dry scaly skin and provides it with moisture. You can create an enriching moisturizer at home by following an easy recipe. Apply this moisturizer on your face daily in the morning or all over your body before taking a bath. It will make your skin smooth, soft and naturally glowing.

Ingredients:

1 cup Buttermilk

½ Avocado

2 Tablespoons of Honey

2-3 drops of Olive Oil

Process:

Mix all the ingredients and grind them. Grind until they start to appear like a lotion. Store it in a bottle. Apply it daily for beautiful glowing skin.

Buttermilk Moisturizer

Buttermilk is one natural ingredient which is high in lactic acid and works like magic for reviving dry scaly skin. It provides the moisture required by the skin and hydrates it. It is said that Queen Cleopatra's secret of beauty was buttermilk.

Dab a cotton ball in the buttermilk and apply it all over your face, neck, and body if required. Don't rub, give it a rest for a while and then wash thoroughly with water. It is easy as that.

Shea Butter Moisturizer

Shea Butter is also commonly known as Shea nut butter. This butter is easily available in the market and provides instant results. It moisturizes your skin and makes it look supple. This butter has healing properties too; it acts as an antiseptic and is effective if used in case of sunburn, eczema and dermatitis.

Olive Oil

Olive oil has numerous benefits; one of which is to moisturize dry skin. Dab a cotton ball in olive oil and apply it to the dry scaly patches on your body or face. Massage the area with tips of fingers and then leave for 5-10 minutes, wash it with warm water afterwards.

Honey

Honey is one integral ingredient in most beauty products. Honey helps in retrieving the moisture of your skin. By massaging your skin with honey, it hydrates your skin and unclogs your pores.

You can make a solution of 1 Tablespoon of honey and 10 Tablespoons of water. Mix well and apply it all over your face. Massage your face and allow it dry and then wash your face with lukewarm water.

General Treatments to Rejuvenate Dry Skin to Achieve Naturally Glowing and Healthy Looking Skin

Apart from all the home remedies mentioned in this eBook there are a few other general remedies for people with dry skin to treat their skin and make it look fresh, supple and hydrated. These home remedies should be at your fingertips at all times.

a. Egg Yolk and Olive Oil

Olive oil is a natural antioxidant and also has vitamin K and E in abundance. These vitamins are essential for all skin types. Whereas egg yolks are enriched with Vitamin A this is the secret for younger looking skin and tightens your skin.

Make a mixture of egg yolk and olive oil and beat them until they form a solution. Apply the solution on your face with the help of a brush and stroke it upwards. The egg yolk will tighten your skin and nourish it with vitamin A. It will remove fine lines and wrinkles whereas olive oil will provide moisture and hydrate your skin. You can even add 2-3 drops of lime water to the solution.

b. Massage with Almond or Coconut Oil

Dry skin loses its moisture; that is why it is patchy and scaly. You can massage your face with almond or coconut oil. It will not only treat the dryness of your skin, but will also moisturize it. The fatty acids present in the coconut oil is very essential for a healthy looking skin, whereas almond oil helps in reviving the moisture of the skin. For best results massage your body with coconut oil before going to bed and wash it off in the morning.

Make sure that you are not allergic to nuts before you start using the oil. People who are allergic to nuts and dry fruits shouldn't use the oil or consult with your doctor first.

c. Banana and Yogurt

Form a mixture of banana and yogurt by mashing banana in yogurt with the help of a fork and then beat it to form a paste. Do not grind or it will get too thin in consistency. Once it is almost a paste apply it all over your face and neck. Allow it to dry then spray rose water on your face and massage your face thoroughly. When it is completely absorbed in your skin, clean your face with the help of a wet cotton ball or a sponge.

You will see a visible difference in your skin right after the first use. You can repeat the procedure 2-3 times a week if your skin is very dry and then reduce the frequency to once a week.

d. Castor Oil

Castor oil is enriched in vitamins and is known for its healing capabilities. The vitamins present in the oil provides its nourishment and hydrates skin during dry weather and in winter.

Herbal Home Remedies for Normal Skin:

Having normal skin means having less trouble than other skin types, but that shouldn't stop you from taking good care of your skin. Because nevertheless, issues like dry patches or an oily T-zone is common with normal skin types as well.

Normal skin isn't very dry or not too oily. It is just normal, as the name suggests. But nothing comes without a price. It definitely takes sincere efforts from your end to keep it glowing and beautiful.

By following a few easy home remedies, you can easily manage to have a glowing, healthy skin. The best part, it's without spending a lot of frequent spa trips or by buying expensive beauty products. Keep these remedies at your fingertips and you will be good to go.

Masks for People with Normal Skin

Tomato and Yogurt Mask:

This mask will help in reducing the effect of sun on your skin and yogurt will serve as an anti-aging agent. It will reduce fine lines and wrinkles.

Ingredients:

1 medium Tomato

2 Tablespoons of Yogurt

Process:

Grind the tomato paste and add yogurt in it and mix well. Apply the mixture to your face and keep massaging gently. Wash your face after 10-15 minutes and apply witch hazel on your face.

Papaya Peel Massage:

Take papaya peel and rub it all over your face. Massage your face with the peel for 5 minutes before washing your face thoroughly with water. Papaya also has antiaging agents. They improve the health of your skin and make it appear glowing.

Egg Mask:

Egg masks works like magic for all skin types; it helps in tightening of the skin, unclogs the pores, and makes your skin look younger.

Take an egg yolk and add 2 Tablespoons of yogurt and apply it to your face. Allow it to dry and remove it with lukewarm water. This mask is for you if you have dry skin patches.

Even normal skin people face aging signs and to cure that nothing works better than an egg white mask. Beat one egg white and then allow the froth to settle. Apply it on your face with upward strokes. Allow the mask to dry and then remove it with lukewarm water. Make sure you constantly massage your face while removing it.

Fuller's Earth and Basil Leaves Mask:

For normal skin people use of a fuller's earth and basil mask made in rose water is the best. It has multiple benefits. It helps you in getting rid of the aging signs, unclogs pores, removes excess oil from your skin and makes it look glowing and healthy.

Ingredients:

1 Tablespoon Fuller's Earth

1 Tablespoon Basil leaves (crushed)

Rose Water

Process:

Make a mixture of all the ingredients and apply it on your face. Allow the mask to dry and then spray rose water on your face. Massage your face with upward strokes and then wash it with water.

Nutmeg and Chickpea Flour Face Mask

Nutmeg is one good old ingredient that is known for being helpful for all skin types in managing healthy looking glowing skin, whereas, chickpea flour has the properties and tendency to absorb excess oil in your skin.

Ingredients:

1 Tablespoon Chickpea Flour Powder

1 Tablespoon nutmeg

Rose Water or Distilled Water

Process:

Mix all the ingredient to form a thick paste. Scrub well on the nose and cheeks. Allow the mask to dry. Then spray rose water on your face and gently massage your face. Remove the mask and wash your face with lukewarm water.

Orange Mask:

Citrus and vitamin C is found in abundance in oranges. It can be used to make normal skin glow and rejuvenate it.

Ingredients:

1½ Tablespoons of Orange Juice

1 Tablespoon of Curd

Process:

Mix the ingredients well and apply the paste on your face as a mask. Allow the mask to dry. Once it is dry sprinkle water or rose water on your face and gently massage your face for 2-3 minutes. Wipe your face firmly with a sponge and wash your face with lukewarm water.

Make Your Toner for Normal Skin At Home:

Toners are an integral to keep your pores closed and keeping any excess oil at bay. Yes even normal skin people often face problems of an oily face. To prevent that, toners help you a lot.

You don't necessarily have to go on a shopping spree to buy the right toners for your skin. You can easily make a toner for normal skin type at home by following these quick recipes.

Cabbage Toner:

Grind cabbage with water or you can even substitute it with rose water. Extract the water from the cabbage and store it in a spray bottle. Apply this toner all over your face after scrubbing or washing your face daily and don't wash afterwards.

Carrot Toner:

Boil baby carrots in water and cook until the color of the water changes. Extract the water and store it in a spray bottle. Use it as toner multiple times a day. Don't wipe it off your face afterwards.

Ice Cubes as Toner:

Lemon grass is not only good for losing weight but they are also good as a toner. Boil lemon grass in a cup of water and then extract the water, keep it aside and allow it to cool. Once it is cool, freeze it in the form of ice cubes. Massage your face daily after washing your face in the morning. Or if possible, massage your face with its ice cubes after being out in sun for several hours.

Herbal Home Remedies to Moisturize Your Skin

Moisturizing your skin is as important as breathing. By reading this eBook you now might have an idea on how important moisturizing your skin is. Your skin is a living being and it requires hydration to look fresh, healthy and glowing.

There are two kinds of moisturizers. One that makes your skin feel soft and supple and the other draws moisture on the epidermis and hydrates it. Usually people with dry skin are complaining about dry and patchy skin. But people with normal and dry skin also need to moisturize their skin. You need to know your skin type to moisturize your skin accordingly.

For instance people with oily skin would need little or no moisturizing but dry and normal skin owners would need to moisturize their skin in order to keep it hydrated and healthy. By keeping these herbal remedies on hand you will be able to moisturize your skin easily at home. Once you try these you will forget you ever used chemical moisturizers.

Quick Herbal Remedies to Moisturize your Skin

Washing your face with soaps and other chemical products can make your skin feel dry. These quick tips will help you keep it supple and moisturized.

a. Goat Milk

After cleansing and scrubbing your face, massage your face with warm goat milk. Yes specifically goat milk. Goat milk lightens your skin tone and gives it natural glow. It also moisturizes your skin.

b. Mashed Bananas

Banana has natural oil. Mash a banana with the help of a fork and add honey if your skin feels extremely dry and patchy. Make a paste and apply it all over your face. Keep massaging your face for a good 10 minutes. Wash your face with lukewarm water.

c. Chocolate

Yes you read it right, a chocolate mask can help you in curing dry skin and moisturizing your skin making it appear supple. Make a yummy mask of chocolate, honey and avocado and you will be surprised by the results.

This mask will not only help you in moisturizing your skin; it will also significantly reduce pimples and blemishes that keep appearing on your skin from time to time. However, don't forget the key factor; clean your face well while removing the mask.

Ingredients:

½ Avocado grinded into small pieces

3 Tablespoons of Melted Dark Chocolate

1 Tablespoon of Honey

Process:

Mix the ingredients in a clean bowl and apply the mixture on your face with the help of a brush. Wear the mask for 10 minutes and then wash your face with lukewarm water.

Herbal Home Remedies To Remove Dark/Brown Spots for Glowing Skin

It is useless to advise someone to avoid sun, you can't live with it and can't live without it. Sun provides us essential vitamins that are a requirement of healthy skin. However, too much exposure to the sun can cause aging and dark or brown spots. These dark spots can also be a result of menopause or pregnancy, weak liver, lack of sun exposure, or Vitamin E as well.

Age/Dark spots make your skin look unappealing and take away the glow from your face. These spots can be termed as liver spots, sunspots or age spots. Whatever you call them; getting rid of these spots is the agenda of the day.

Getting rid of these dark spots isn't difficult at all. However you will be required to do a little care and follow these simple home remedies that suits your skin type to get rid of these dark spots and regain your flawless glowing skin.

Easy Remedies You Can Follow At Home

It is essential to figure out the reason of these dark spots. However general herbal and home remedies in this eBook will help just about everyone.

Lemon Juice

Extract fresh lemon juice and apply it on the dark patches and spots. Give it a rest for about 30 minutes. Don't itch or rub it. Wash your face with lukewarm water after 30 minutes.

If you have dark spots on your face, then applying lemon juice directly will do for you. Avoid doing it if you have acne. Dilute it with rose water and then apply. For dark spots on hands, arms and legs, rub lemon peel directly on the dark spots. You will see visible results right after the first use.

Sandalwood

Sandalwood has many benefits for skin. It helps in skin tone lightening and is also extremely useful for getting rid of age and brown spots. Face mask and home remedies that involve Sandalwood are easy to apply and highly effective.

Ingredients:

2 Tablespoons of Sandalwood powder

1 Tablespoon of Glycerin

1 Tablespoon of Rose Water

Process:

Make a face mask by mixing all these ingredients. Apply the mixture on your face and allow it dry. Wash your face after 30 minutes with cold water. It is advised that you do it at least once a day for a week.

Sandalwood oil can also serve as an extremely effective herbal remedy. Apply sandalwood oil directly on the affected area and massage gently. Do this daily for a week and then 2-3 times a week after that. You will see visible results.

Onion and Garlic:
Use of Onion and Garlic on dark spots also helps in removing dark spots and aging signs.

Ingredients:

1 Onion

2-3 cloves of Garlic

Process:

Extract the juice of onion and garlic. Mix them together and form a solution. Apply on the dark spots and leave it for about 10-15 minutes. Wash your face thoroughly and apply rose water on your face. This will remove the smell of onion and garlic from your face.

This mixture is highly effective when it comes to reducing and eventually removing dark and brown spots.

Onion:

You can also reduce these dark spots by rubbing onion directly on the dark spot. Gently rub the onion. Your skin might start feeling itchy if you rub it vigorously.

Horseradish
Horseradish if combined with other essential ingredients can be very effective as well.

Ingredients:

2-3 Tablespoons of Horseradish (Grated)

1 Tablespoon of Lemon Juice

1 Tablespoon of Vinegar

1 Tablespoon of Rosemary Oil

Few drops of Olive Oil

Process:

Mix all the ingredients and form a paste. Apply the mixture on your face or the dark spots. Rub the horseradish from the solution on the dark spots and leave it for 15-20 minutes. Wipe your face with the help of a sponge and then wash your face thoroughly with lukewarm or warm water.

It is advised to apply this solution on your face once or twice a day daily to get rid of the dark or aging spots.

Buttermilk:

Buttermilk is very effective when it comes to skin care. It is extremely helpful for removing makeup and blackheads. It is also helpful in getting rid of dark spots and aging signs.

Apply buttermilk on the dark spots before going to bed. Massage gently. Wash the area in the morning with warm water. Make this a habit before going to bed. This will not only reduce dark spots but will also prevent dark spots from appearing on your skin.

Red Currants

This remedy is as yummy as the fruit itself. You will have to resist your temptation to eat the fruit if you want to cure the dark spots. Ok may be you can have a few.

Ingredients:

2 Tablespoons of Unripe Red currants (Mashed)

1 Tablespoon Honey

Process:

Make a mixture of the ingredients and make a paste. Mix well until the mixture is of uniform consistency. Apply the mixture as a mask on your skin. Not to mention the appealing aroma, the mixture will calm your senses and will reduce dark spots and lighten your skin tone.

You can wash your face with lukewarm water and then apply rose water as a toner. This remedy can also be applied to other affected areas like on arms and legs.

There is another extremely easy remedy that is very useful in removing dark spots:

Ingredients:

1 Tablespoon of Red currant pulp

2 Tablespoon of Orange Juice

1 Tablespoon of Parsley

1 Tablespoon of Lemon Juice

Process:

Make a mixture of all the ingredients and make a paste. Apply the paste on the dark spots and massage gently. Leave it for 10-15 minutes and wash thoroughly with lukewarm water.

Sugar

Sugar is highly effective for moisturizing your skin. It can also help you in getting rid of dark spots and aging signs.

Take equal portions of white and brown sugar. Add enough rose water to make a paste. Dissolve the sugar in the rose water as much as you can. Apply the syrup on the affected areas and massage well. Wash your hands with lukewarm water and apply lemon juice or massage for another 5 minutes with lemon peel for best results.

Fruit Treatment for Brown/Dark Spots:

Apricot and Strawberry Paste

You may be familiar with the wonders of apricot. It makes a very good scrub and helps in getting rid of various skin problems. Apricot, if combined with strawberry can be very effective for most of your skin problems. Strawberry has citrus and other essential natural elements that are required by your skin. You can use this paste as a mask as well.

Ingredients:

½ Apricot

2-3 Strawberries

Process:

Mash or grind the ingredients and form a pulp. If it is too dry add 1 Tablespoon of rose water or honey. Apply this paste on the affected areas and massage well. Leave it on your skin for 10-20 minutes and then wash thoroughly with water.

Watermelon

Watermelon has a soothing effect on skin. Face masks that contain watermelon leaves your skin fresh and glowing. Watermelon if combined with grains of rice can do wonders for your skin. This includes removing and reducing dark spots, wrinkles and other signs of aging.

Ingredients:

1 bowl of freshly cut watermelon

2-3 Tablespoon of Rice Grains

Process:

Put the rice with the watermelon and store it in the fridge for the whole night. The rice will get soaked and swell by the morning. Grind or mash the rice and watermelon and make a pulp like mixture of it. Apply the mixture on the affected area and leave if for 10-20 minutes. Wipe off the contents and wash your skin thoroughly with water.

Papaya

Papaya is a key ingredient of many beauty products that you use on the daily basis. Little did you know that using this fruit directly instead of in the form of chemical products will yield more effective and prompt results.

Here are a couple of ways by which you can reduce dark spots and aging signs using papaya.

a. Rub the papaya peel directly on the dark spots for 5-10 minutes. Do it once or twice a week.
b. Massage the affected area with papaya juice. Repeat the procedure daily before going to bed and wash your skin thoroughly the next morning.

Apple Cider Vinegar

Apple cider vinegar mixed with onion juice is also one of the many effective herbal home remedies you can count on. Apply the mixture on your skin for 10-15 minutes. This will have visible effects on the dark spots and aging signs.

Take equal portions of Onion extract and apple cider vinegar, preferably 1 Tablespoon of each ingredient for one time use. It is advised to make a fresh solution every time.

Herbal Remedies to Polish Your Skin for Natural Glow

What you can achieve by frequent spa visits, you can get easily at home without a hassle. To gain a healthy glowing skin, skin polishing also plays a pivotal role. Strict working hours, hectic routines, sun exposure and pollution can take away the shine from your face making it appear dull and dry.

We all know the hefty amount that any one will have to pay if they want to go for a full body polish at the local spa. However with these quick herbal home remedies, you can polish your skin at home within no time at a significantly reduced price.

It is integral to know your skin type when it comes to skin polishing. If you have dry and sensitive skin, oily or normal. You need to determine that before opting for any of the skin polishing methods mentioned in this eBook. Here are some all natural and herbal methods that you can use to polish your skin.

Body Polish According to Skin Type

Oily Skin

Body polish ingredients like sea salt and other minerals works like magic for oily skin people. They not only help in oil controlling but give your skin a natural shine and glow that is not because of oil.

Normal Skin

Having a normal skin complexion is like winning the lottery. Sugar, rice, apricot, avocados, coffee, etc. There are gazillions of choices available for people with normal skin types to choose from.

Dry Skin

For dry skin you can opt for a body polish that has soft ingredients. Ingredients like Sandalwood powder, Aromatic Flower Oils, Avocado, Brown Sugar and geranium. These ingredients are ideal for people with dry skin. The task of the ingredients is to properly hydrate your skin and polish it for a glowing effect.

Sensitive Skin

People with sensitive skin should opt for a body polish with moist ingredients and not the ones which have dry chunks like apricot. Go with ingredients like Shea butter, cocoa butter with Lavender or Chamomile aromatic oils. These aromatic oils have soothing and calming effects on your body and skin and can also relax your mind.

Body Polishes

Sea Salt Body Polish
Ingredients:

1 Cup Sea Salt

4 Tablespoons of Aloe Vera Gel

2 Tablespoons of Lavender oil

2 Tablespoons of Essential Tea Tree Oil

½ Tablespoons of Olive Oil

Process:

Mix all the ingredients well and mash the Aloe Vera gel if needed. Form a semi paste mixture and apply it all over your hands, legs, face, and neck. Allow the face and neck to dry while you massage your hands and feet and absorb the ingredients as much as you can into your skin. Then massage your face specially emphasizing on the nose, chin, cheeks and forehead. Give it a rest for about 30 minutes and then take a hot water bath.

Brown Sugar Body Polish
Ingredients:

6 Tablespoons of Brown Sugar

6 Tablespoons of Olive Oil

3 Tablespoons of Oatmeal

Process:

Mix all the ingredients together and form a solution. Apply the solution all over your body and massage well. While massaging your face, make sure you focus on the nose and cheeks. Allow yourself to enjoy the luxury of a hot water bath afterwards.

Conclusion

Herbal remedies have been among us for centuries. People have been using them for curing different ailments. Herbal remedies as compared to chemical beauty products are extremely useful and have little or no side effects. It is however advised that you consult your doctor before applying anything. Don't forget to keep in mind if you are allergic to any natural or herbal product.

Some herbal medicines mentioned in this eBook would start showing quick and immediate results however you will have to be patient with others. Because these remedies takes their time before they start showing results.

Using herbal tips and home remedies to have a naturally beautiful, glowing and healthy skin is the best and effective way. Herbal remedies have significantly less side effects compared to the beauty products and treatments available in the market.

www.ingramcontent.com/pod-product-compliance
Lightning Source LLC
Chambersburg PA
CBHW052019280526
45793CB00005B/1046